TITLE:

BASIC DAILY WEIGHT LOSS EXERCISE.

Subtitle:

15 Minutes to a Slimmer You

JOSEPH V. GOODING

ABOUT THE AUTHOR

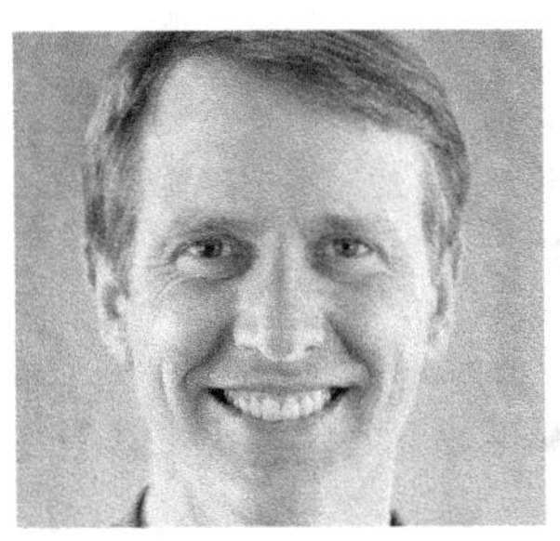 **JOSEPH V. GOODING** is a Fitness Instructor and among a passionate group of certified personal trainers, registered dietitians, and exercise physiologists dedicated to helping people achieve their weight loss and fitness goals.

With over [15] years of combined experience, He has helped countless individuals transform their lives by creating safe, effective, and sustainable exercise routines.

His mission is to empower people of all fitness levels to embrace a healthy lifestyle through accessible daily exercise programs.

He believes that weight loss should be a journey, not a punishment, and He is here to guide and support you every step of the way.

TABLE OF CONTENTS

Part 1:

The Foundation of Daily Exercise for Weight Loss

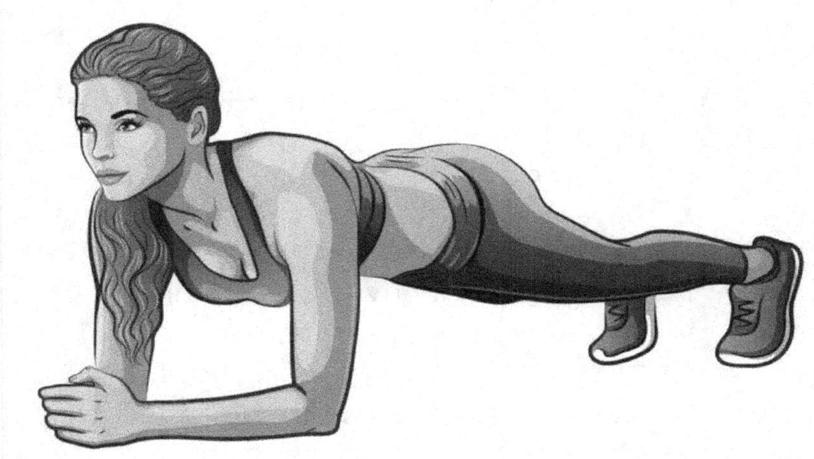

Chapter 1: Introduction

Welcome to your transformation! This book is your roadmap to shedding pounds and building a healthier you through the power of daily exercise. Whether you're a complete beginner or looking to jumpstart a weight loss routine, this guide provides a foundation for sustainable success.

Why Daily Exercise Matters for Weight Loss:

- **Boosts Metabolism:** Regular physical activity elevates your metabolic rate, meaning your body burns more calories throughout the day, even at rest.
- **Burns Fat:** Exercise directly targets fat stores, helping you shed unwanted weight and sculpt a more toned physique.
- **Improves Mood and Energy:** Physical activity releases endorphins, natural mood-lifters that combat stress and fatigue, leaving you feeling energized and motivated.
- **Builds Muscle:** Strength training builds muscle mass, which further increases your metabolism and helps maintain a healthy weight.

- **Strengthens Your Heart:** Regular exercise keeps your heart healthy and reduces your risk of cardiovascular disease.

What to Expect in This Book:

This book dives into the world of basic daily weight loss exercises. It will equip you with:

- **Simple and effective exercises:** We'll explore a variety of bodyweight exercises and light equipment routines that require minimal space and no gym membership.
- **Daily workout plans:** We'll provide flexible daily exercise plans tailored to different fitness levels, allowing you to customize your routine based on your needs and preferences.
- **Essential exercise techniques:** You'll learn proper form and technique to ensure you maximize results and avoid injury.
- **Motivation and tips:** We'll offer valuable guidance to stay motivated, overcome challenges, and integrate exercise seamlessly into your daily life.

Embrace the Journey:

This book is your companion on your weight loss journey through daily exercise. *Remember, consistency is key. It's not about pushing yourself to exhaustion every day, but about creating a sustainable routine you can enjoy and maintain in the long term. Let's get started on building a healthier, happier you, one exercise at a time!*

Chapter 2: Understanding Weight Loss and the Role of Exercise:

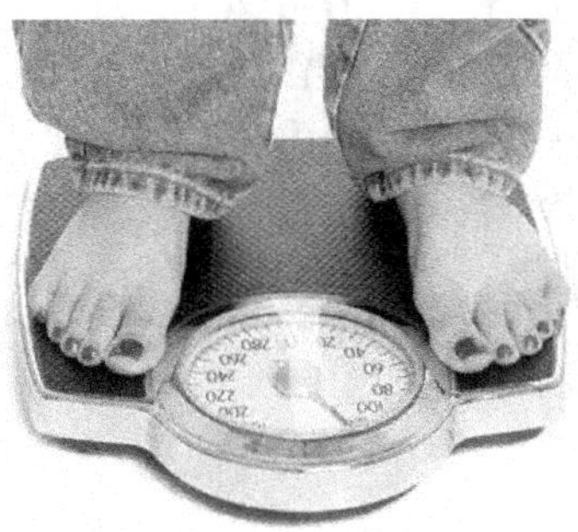

Welcome to the science behind your weight loss journey! This chapter dives into the core principles that will guide your success: calorie balance, healthy eating, and the power of different types of exercise.

Calories In vs. Calories Out:

Imagine your body as a bank account for energy. You deposit energy through the food and drinks you consume (calories in). You withdraw energy through daily activities and exercise (calories out). Weight loss boils down to having a calorie deficit, meaning you burn more calories than you consume.

- Calories: These are units of energy that your body uses to function.
- Basal Metabolic Rate (BMR): This is the

number of calories your body burns at rest, just to maintain its basic functions like breathing and circulation.
- Activity Level: The calories you burn through daily activities like walking, working, and exercising.

The Importance of Combining Exercise with Healthy Eating:

Simply burning more calories than you consume is key, but what you eat matters too. Here's why:

- Healthy Eating Fuels Your Workouts: Nutritious foods provide the energy you need to power through your workouts and support muscle recovery. Junk food leaves you feeling sluggish and hinders your weight loss efforts.
- Nutrient Deficiencies: A poor diet can lead to nutrient deficiencies that affect your metabolism and overall health.
- Muscle Building: Building muscle mass through strength training increases your metabolism, helping you burn more calories even at rest. However, muscle needs protein to grow and repair itself.

Types of Exercise and Their Impact on Weight Loss:

Exercise plays a crucial role in creating a calorie deficit and boosting weight loss. Let's explore two main types:

- Cardio (Aerobic Exercise): Cardio activities like brisk walking, running, swimming, or cycling elevate your heart rate and increase your breathing. They are fantastic for burning calories during the workout.

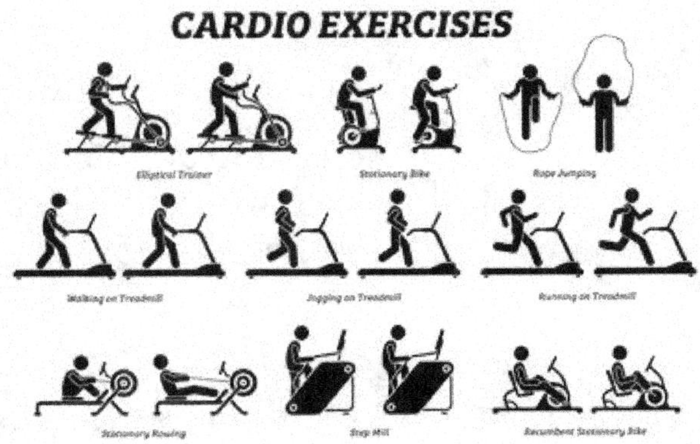

- Strength Training: Lifting weights or using bodyweight exercises builds muscle mass. Muscle burns more calories than fat, even at rest, contributing to a higher metabolism and increased calorie burning throughout the day.

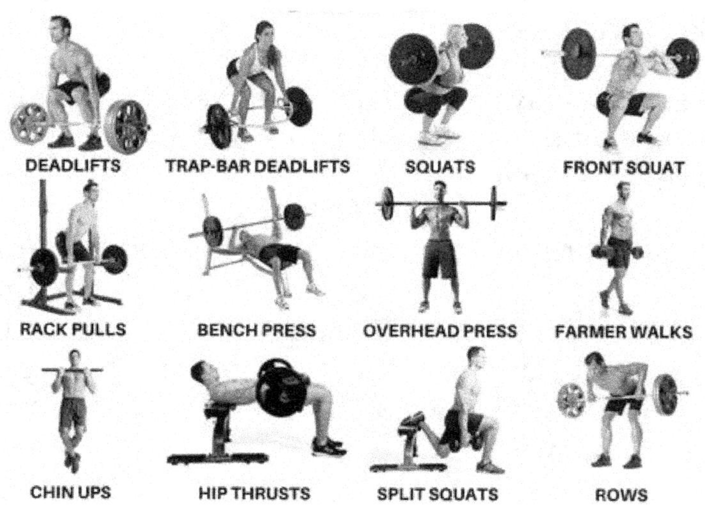

How Each Type Contributes to Weight Loss:

- Cardio: Burns a significant amount of calories during the workout, ideal for creating a calorie deficit.

- Strength Training: Builds muscle mass, which boosts your metabolism and increases calorie burning throughout the day, even at rest. It also helps you maintain muscle while losing fat, leading to a more toned physique.

The Ideal Combination:

For optimal weight loss, combine both cardio and strength training. Cardio helps you burn calories quickly, while strength training builds muscle and boosts your metabolism for long-term benefits.

Chapter 3: Getting Started with Daily Exercise:

Congratulations on taking the first step towards a healthier you! This chapter equips you with essential tips specifically designed for beginners to kickstart your daily exercise routine safely and effectively.

Setting Realistic Goals:

Setting ambitious goals is great, but starting small and gradually increasing intensity is key to long-term success. Here's how to set realistic goals:

Focus on Habits, Not Numbers: Instead of aiming to lose 10 pounds in a month, aim to exercise for 20 minutes daily. This builds a sustainable habit.

Start Small and Gradually Increase: Begin with short, manageable workouts and gradually increase duration and intensity as your fitness improves.

Celebrate Milestones: Acknowledge and celebrate your progress, no matter how small. This keeps you motivated and on track.

Choosing Comfortable Workout Gear:

The right attire can make a world of difference in your workout experience. Here's what to consider:

Comfortable Clothing: Choose breathable, loose-fitting clothes that allow for freedom of movement. Avoid restrictive clothing or cotton that gets heavy with sweat.

Supportive Shoes: Invest in a good pair of athletic shoes that provide proper support and cushioning for your chosen activities.

Warming Up and Cooling Down:

These routines prepare your body for exercise and aid in recovery, preventing injuries and muscle soreness.

Warm-Up (5-10 minutes): Light cardio like jumping jacks, jogging in place, or arm circles increases blood flow and warms up your muscles.

Cool-Down (5-10 minutes): Gentle stretches hold for 20-30 seconds each to improve flexibility and prevent post-workout stiffness.

Listen to Your Body:

Your body is your best guide. Here's how to listen to its signals:

Pay Attention to Pain: Pain is different from discomfort. If you experience sharp pain, stop the exercise and consult a doctor before continuing.

Take Rest Days: Rest allows your body to recover and repair muscle tissue. Aim for at least one rest day per week.

Modify Exercises: Don't be afraid to modify exercises to suit your fitness level. There are always easier variations you can do until you progress.

Preventing Injuries:

By following these tips, you can significantly reduce your risk of injuries:

Proper Form: Focus on proper form during exercises to avoid straining muscles or joints. Don't hesitate to ask a trainer or gym staff for guidance if needed.

Don't Push Yourself Too Hard: Start slowly and gradually increase intensity. Pushing yourself beyond your limits increases the risk of injuries.

Stay Hydrated: Drink plenty of water before, during, and after your workouts to stay hydrated and prevent muscle cramps.

Chapter 4: Building a Sustainable Exercise Routine:

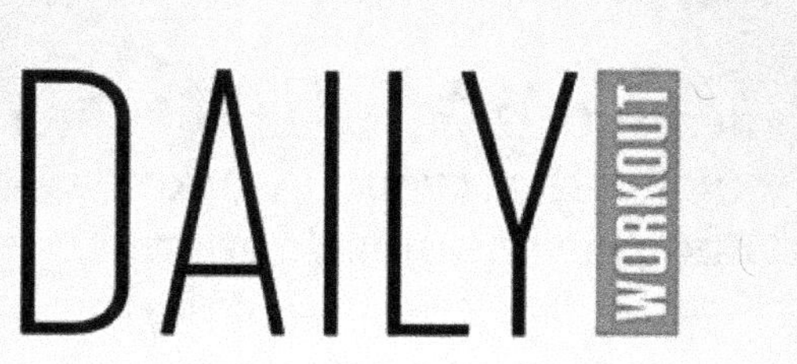

Creating a sustainable daily exercise routine is the key to unlocking long-term weight loss success. This chapter equips you with strategies to seamlessly integrate exercise into your busy life, overcome common challenges, and build a lifelong habit of movement.

Integrating Exercise into Your Schedule:

Find Your Exercise Time: Identify a time that works best for you, whether it's mornings before work, lunchtime breaks, or evenings. Consistency is more important than the time itself.

Schedule It In: Treat your workouts like important appointments and block them off on your calendar. This helps you prioritize exercise and avoid scheduling conflicts.

Start Small and Build Up: Begin with short, manageable workouts and gradually increase duration and intensity as your fitness improves. Even 10-minute bursts of activity make a difference.

Combine Activities: Sneak in exercise throughout your day. Take the stairs instead of the elevator, park farther away from your destination, or do bodyweight exercises during commercial breaks while watching TV.

Overcoming Common Challenges:

Lack of Time: Even the busiest schedules can accommodate exercise. Here are some tips:

a)   High-Intensity Interval Training (HIIT): Short bursts of intense exercise followed by rest periods offer a time-efficient workout with significant calorie burn.

b)   Morning Workouts: Start your day energized with a quick exercise routine before work.

c)   Multitasking: Listen to audiobooks or podcasts while walking, jogging, or cycling.

Lack of Motivation: Motivation can fluctuate. Here's how to stay fired up:

a) Find Activities You Enjoy: Explore different types of exercise until you find activities you genuinely enjoy. This makes staying consistent much easier.

b) Set Achievable Goals: Set realistic goals that celebrate progress and keep you motivated. Reward yourself for reaching milestones.

c) Find a Workout Buddy: Exercising with a friend or family member can boost accountability and make workouts more fun.

Creating a Habit of Exercise:

Making exercise a habit takes time and effort. Here are some strategies:

Focus on Consistency: Aim for consistency over intensity. Even short, daily workouts are more effective in the long run than sporadic bursts of intense exercise.

Track Your Progress: Use a fitness tracker, journal, or app to monitor your progress.

Seeing your improvement is a great motivator.

Celebrate Milestones: Acknowledge and celebrate your achievements, no matter how small. This reinforces the positive association with exercise.

Reward Yourself: Set healthy rewards for reaching goals, like a new workout outfit or a relaxing massage.

Staying Consistent in the Long Run:

Maintaining a consistent exercise routine requires dedication, but the benefits are well worth it. Here are some tips for long-term success:

Find an Exercise Support System: Surround yourself with positive influences who encourage your fitness goals.

Make it Fun: Explore new exercise routines, classes, or activities to keep things interesting and prevent boredom.

Focus on How You Feel: Shift your focus from weight loss to the positive feelings exercise brings, like increased energy, improved mood, and stress reduction.

Forgive Yourself for Setbacks: Everyone experiences setbacks. Don't let a missed workout derail your progress. Just get back on track with your next scheduled session.

By incorporating all the strategies mentioned in part one, you'll transform your daily exercise routine from a chore into a sustainable habit that fuels your weight loss journey and overall well-being for years to come.

Part 2

Daily Exercise Routines for Weight Loss

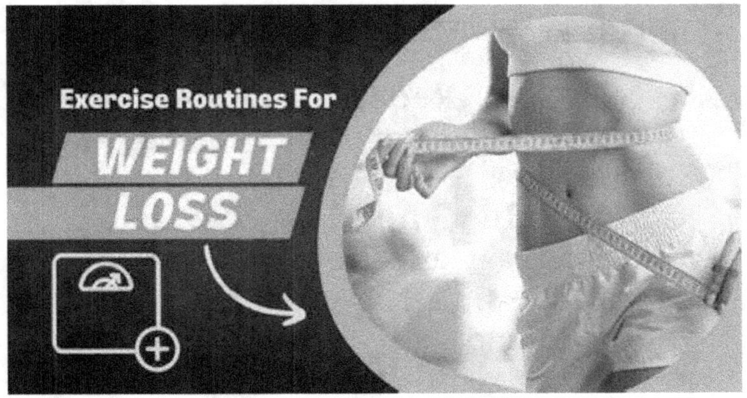

Chapter 5: Daily Workouts for Beginners:

This chapter equips you with a beginner-friendly arsenal of bodyweight exercises that require minimal equipment and can be done anywhere. We'll provide clear instructions, modifications for different fitness levels, and sample daily workout routines to kickstart your weight loss journey.

Benefits of Bodyweight Exercises:

- **No Gym Required:** These exercises require no equipment, making them perfect for home workouts.
- **Adaptable for All Levels:** Most bodyweight exercises can be modified to suit your fitness level, making them ideal for beginners.
- **Engage Multiple Muscle Groups:** Many bodyweight exercises work various muscle groups, providing a well-rounded workout.

Mastering the Basics:

Here are some essential bodyweight exercises with clear instructions and modifications:

1. Squats:

- **Instructions:** Stand with feet shoulder-width apart, toes slightly outward. Lower your body as if sitting in a chair, keeping your back straight and core engaged. Push through your heels to return to standing.
- **Modification (Beginner):** Perform a squat against a wall for support.

2. Lunges:

- **Instructions:** Step forward with one leg, lowering your hips until both knees are bent at 90-degree angles. Push through your front heel to return to standing and repeat with the other leg.
- **Modification (Beginner):** Start with a smaller lunge step or perform stationary lunges without stepping forward.

3. Push-Ups (Modification: Wall Push-Ups):

- **Instructions (Wall Push-Ups):** Stand facing a wall, arms shoulder-width apart, hands flat on the wall. Lean into the wall, keeping your body in a straight line from head to heels, and bend your elbows to lower your chest towards the wall. Push back up to the starting position.
- **Modification (Beginner):** Perform push-ups on your knees instead of your toes.

4. Plank:

- **Instructions:** Get into a high plank position on your forearms, elbows shoulder-width apart, and body in a straight line from head to heels. Engage your core and glutes to hold the position.
- **Modification (Beginner):** Perform a plank on your knees instead of your forearms.

Sample Daily Workout Routines for Beginners:

Workout A:

- Warm-up: 5 minutes of light cardio (jumping jacks, jogging in place) and dynamic stretches.

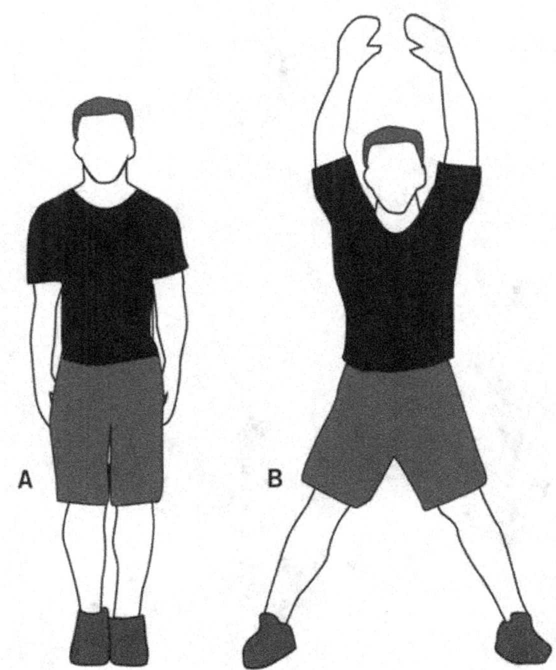

Cool-down: 5 minutes of static stretches focusing on major muscle groups.

10 Bodyweight Squats (3 sets)

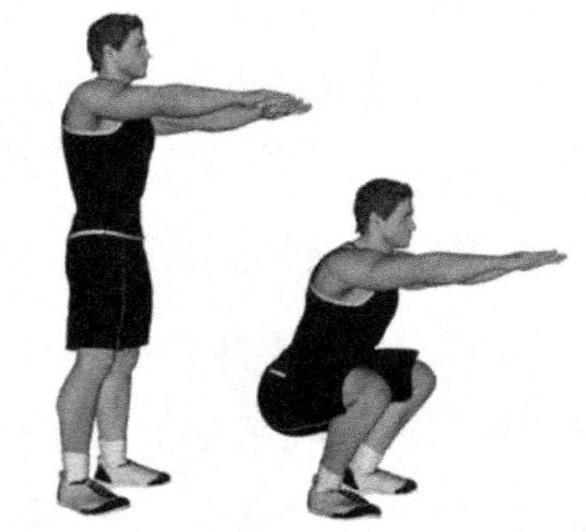

A

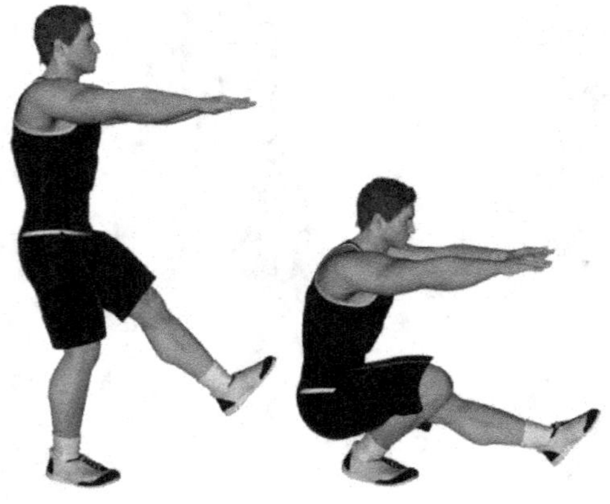

B

Sample Daily Workout Routines for Beginners:

Workout A:

- Warm-up: 5 minutes of light cardio (jumping jacks, jogging in place) and dynamic stretches.

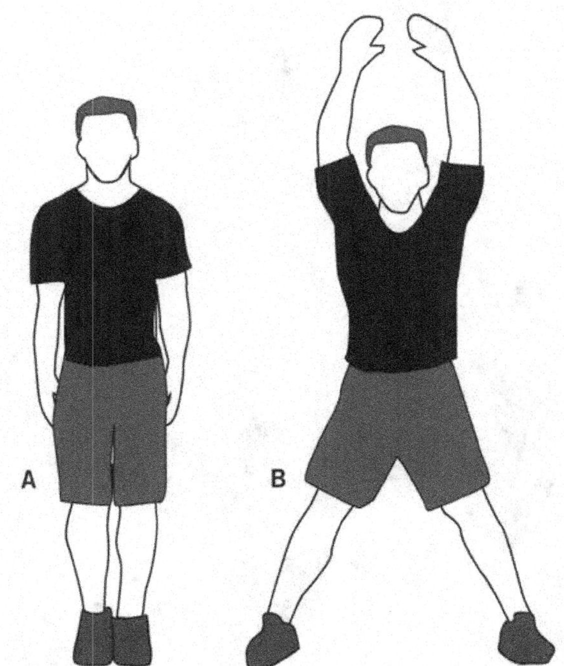

Cool-down: 5 minutes of static stretches focusing on major muscle groups.

10 Bodyweight Squats (3 sets)

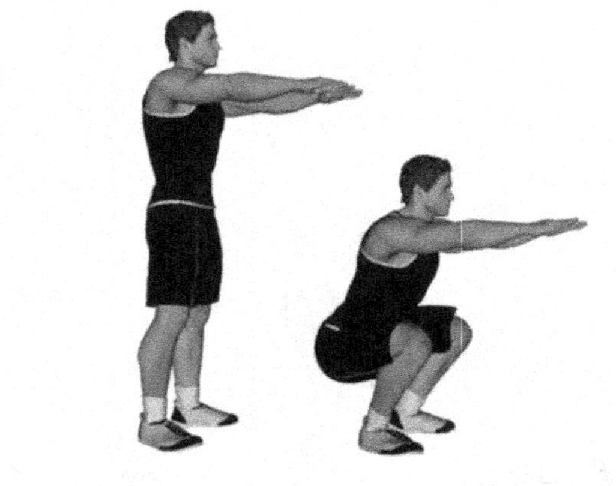

A

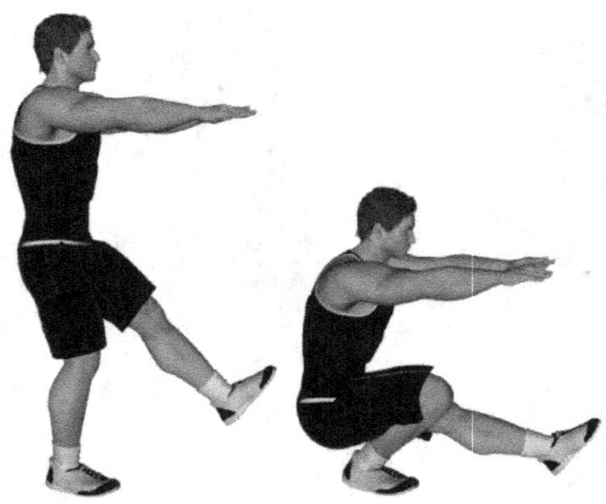

B

Cool-down: 5 minutes of static stretches focusing on major muscle groups.

• **8 Walking Lunges per leg (3 sets)**

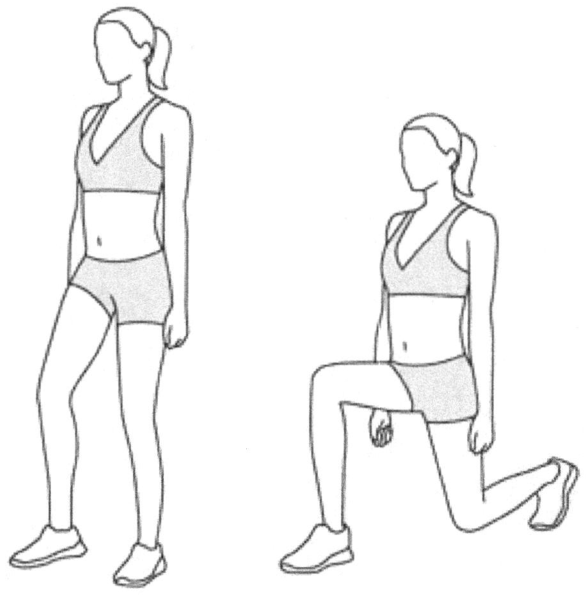

Cool-down: 5 minutes of static stretches focusing on major muscle groups.

- **10 Wall Push-Ups (3 sets)**

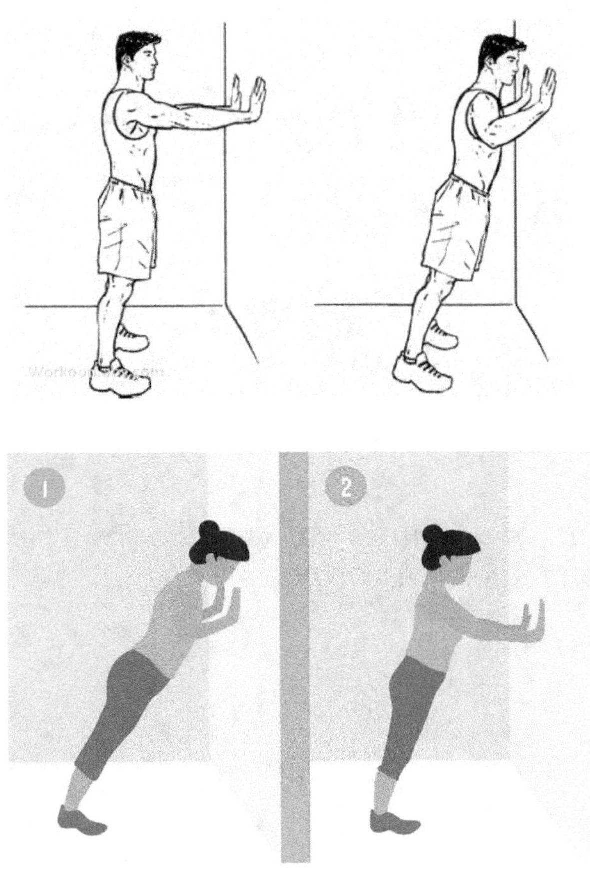

Cool-down: 5 minutes of static stretches focusing on major muscle groups.

- **30-second Plank (3 sets)**

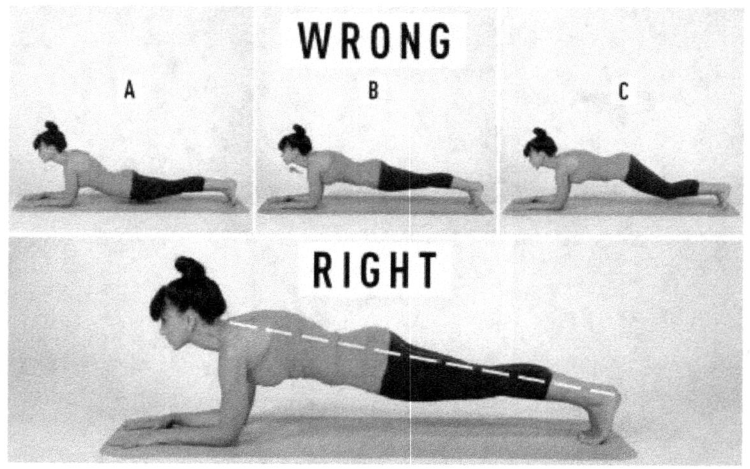

Cool-down: 5 minutes of static stretches focusing on major muscle groups.

Workout B:

- Warm-up (same as Workout A).
- 12 Bodyweight Squats (3 sets)
- 10 Stationary Lunges per leg (3 sets)
- Knee Push-Ups (3 sets of as many repetitions as possible)
- 45-second Plank (3 sets)
- Cool-down (same as Workout A).

Remember:

- Rest for 30 seconds between sets and 1 minute between exercises.
- Focus on proper form over the number of repetitions.
- As you get stronger, increase the number of repetitions, sets, or hold time for each exercise.

These are just a few examples. Feel free to mix and match these exercises to create your own personalized daily workout routines. With consistent effort, you'll build strength, improve endurance, and be well on your way to achieving your weight loss goals!

Chapter 6: Leveling Up Your Daily Workouts:

Congratulations on your progress! You've mastered the basics of bodyweight exercises. This chapter introduces light equipment and more challenging bodyweight exercises to elevate your daily workouts, increase intensity, and build more muscle for enhanced calorie burning and weight loss.

Benefits of Light Equipment:

Increased Intensity: Dumbbells and resistance bands add resistance, making exercises more challenging and helping you build muscle faster.

Targets Specific Muscle Groups: Light equipment allows you to target specific muscle groups for a more sculpted physique.

Affordable and Versatile: Dumbbells and resistance bands are relatively inexpensive and offer a variety of exercise options.

Introducing Light Equipment:

Dumbbells: Start with lighter weights (2-5 lbs) and gradually increase as you get stronger. Choose weights that challenge you for the last 2-3 repetitions of each set.

Resistance Bands: These come in various resistance levels. Choose bands that provide enough tension to challenge you throughout the exercise.

Sample Bodyweight Exercises for Intermediate Levels:

Squats with Dumbbells: Hold dumbbells at shoulder level while performing regular squats.

Walking Lunges with Overhead Press: Hold dumbbells overhead while performing walking lunges.

Decline Push-Ups: Perform push-ups with your feet elevated on a bench or chair for a more challenging variation.

Dips: Use a sturdy chair or bench to perform dips, engaging your triceps and chest muscles.

Light Equipment Exercises:

Dumbbell Rows: Targets your back muscles. Hinge at the hips, keeping your back straight, and row the dumbbells towards your chest.

Dumbbell Overhead Press: Works your shoulders and triceps. Press the dumbbells overhead until your arms are straight.

Bicep Curls: Isolates your biceps. Curl the dumbbells towards your shoulders while keeping your elbows close to your body.

Resistance Band Chest Flyes: Targets your chest muscles. Hold the resistance band in front of you with your arms extended and perform a fly motion, bringing your hands together.

Sample Daily Workout Routines for Intermediate Exercisers:

Workout A:

- **Warm-up (5 minutes of light cardio and dynamic stretches).**

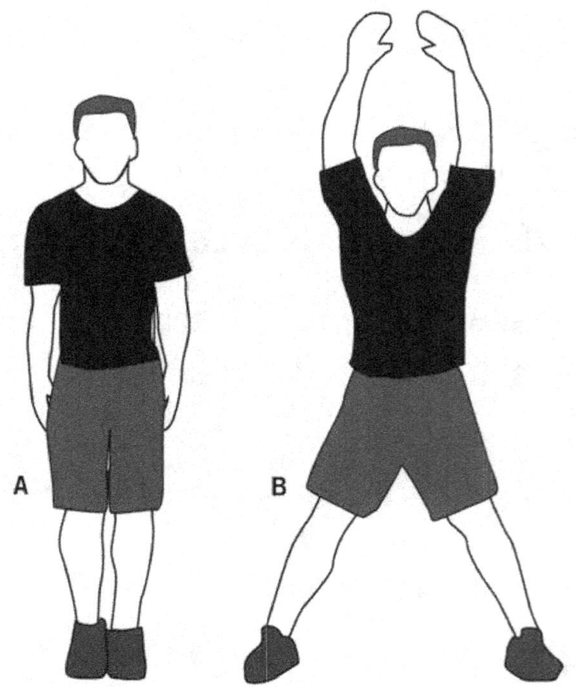

- ## 12 Dumbbell Squats (3 sets)

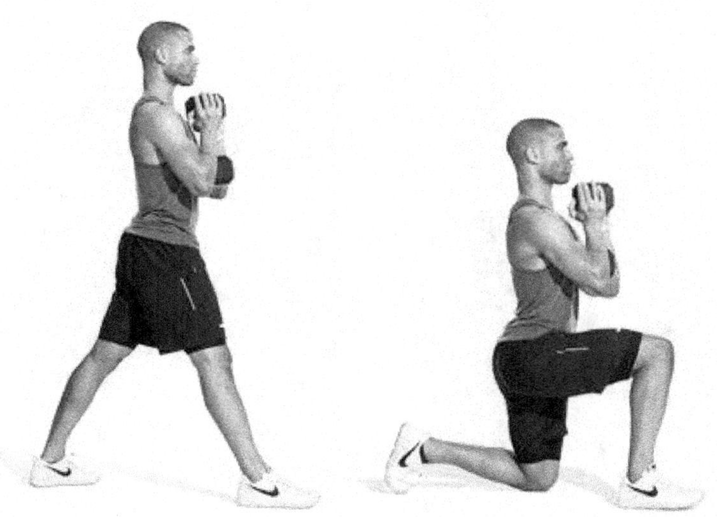

- **10 Walking Lunges with Overhead Press per leg (3 sets)**

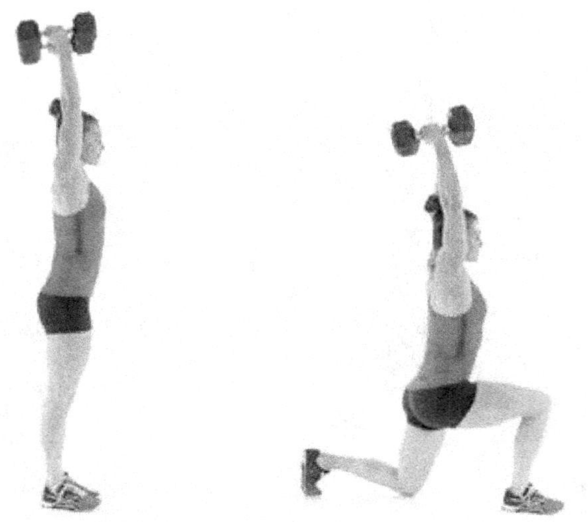

• **8 Decline Push-Ups (3 sets)**

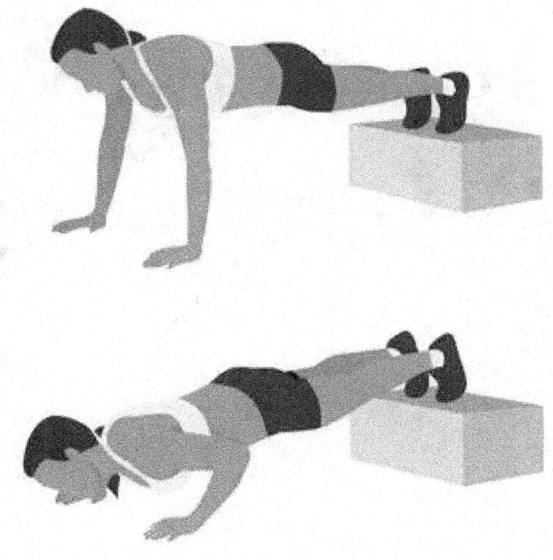

• 10 Dumbbell Rows (3 sets)

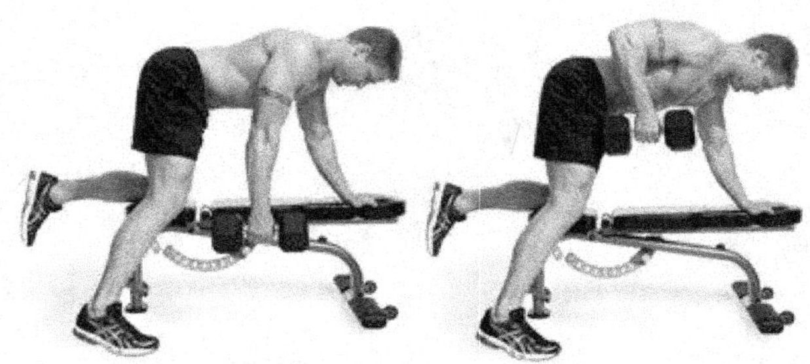

• **10 Dumbbell Overhead Press (3 sets)**

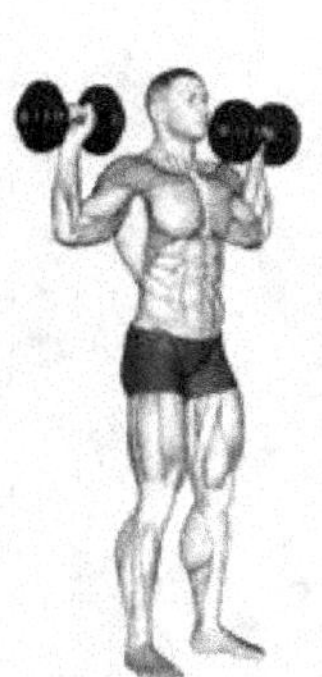 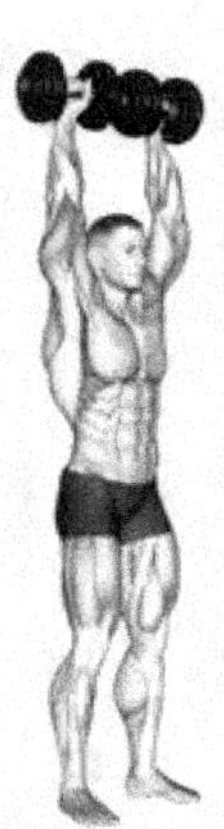

• **12 Bicep Curls (3 sets)**

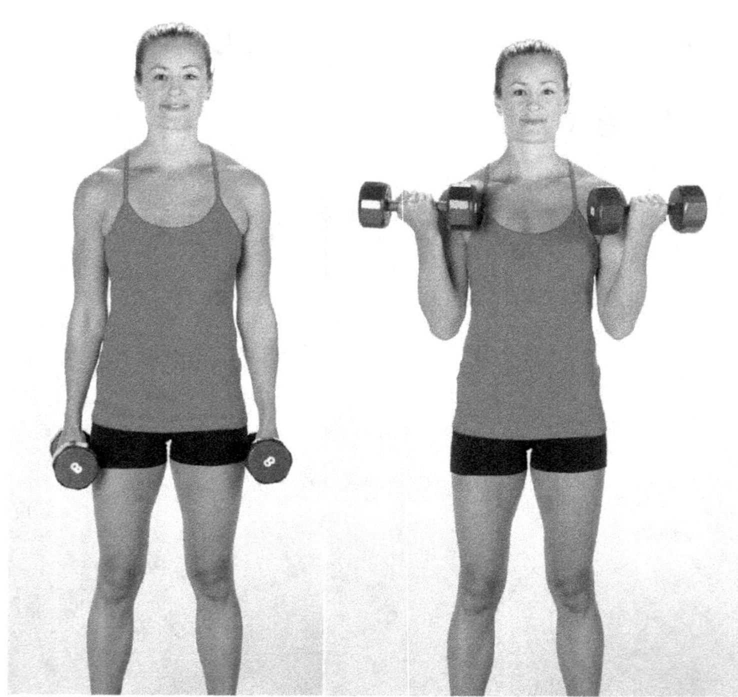

- **3 x 30-second Resistance Band Chest Flyes (3 sets)**

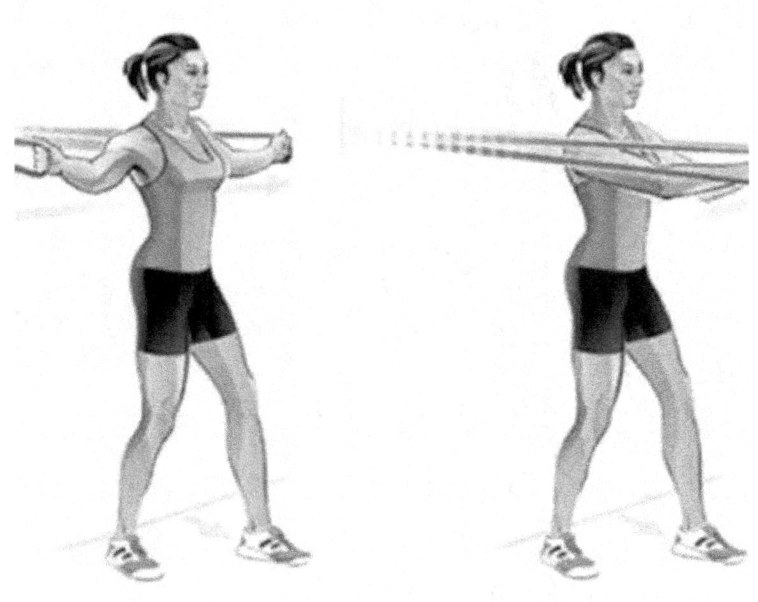

- **Cool-down (5 minutes of static stretches).**

Workout B:

- Warm-up (same as Workout A).
- 15 Dumbbell Squats (3 sets)
- 12 Walking Lunges per leg (3 sets)

- Dips (3 sets of as many repetitions as possible)
- 12 Dumbbell Rows (3 sets)
- 12 Dumbbell Overhead Press (3 sets)
- 15 Bicep Curls (3 sets)
- 3 x 45-second Resistance Band Chest Flyes (3 sets)
- Cool-down (same as Workout A).

Remember:

- As you get stronger, increase the weight of the dumbbells, the resistance of the bands, or the number of sets and repetitions.
- Maintain proper form throughout the exercises.
- Listen to your body and take rest days when needed.

By incorporating light equipment and challenging bodyweight exercises into your daily routine, you'll torch more calories, build muscle, and progress towards your weight loss goals at a faster pace!

Chapter 7: Daily Workouts for Different Fitness Goals:

You've come a long way! Now, let's tailor your daily workouts to your specific fitness goals. This chapter provides targeted routines for building muscle, improving cardiovascular health, burning belly fat, and increasing flexibility.

Building Muscle:

Focus: Compound exercises that work multiple muscle groups simultaneously.

Sample Daily Routine:

- Warm-up (5 minutes of light cardio and dynamic stretches).
- Squats with Dumbbells (3 sets of 8-12 repetitions)
- Dumbbell Rows (3 sets of 8-12 repetitions)
- Push-Ups (Decline or Wall Push-Ups if needed) (3 sets of as many repetitions as possible)
- Overhead Press (Dumbbells or Bodyweight) (3 sets of 8-12 repetitions)

- ○ Rest for 1-2 minutes between sets.
- ○ Cool-down (5 minutes of static stretches).

Progression: Increase weight, sets, or repetitions as you get stronger.

Improving Cardiovascular Fitness:

- **Focus:** Cardio exercises that elevate your heart rate and sustain it for an extended period.
- **Sample Daily Routine:**
  - ○ Warm-up (5 minutes of light cardio).
  - ○ 30 minutes of Brisk Walking, Running, Swimming, Cycling, or Jumping Rope.
  - ○ Maintain a moderate intensity where you can hold a conversation but breathing is slightly labored.
  - ○ Cool-down (5 minutes of light cardio and static stretches).
- **Progression:** Gradually increase the duration or intensity of your cardio workouts.

Burning Belly Fat:

- **Focus:** A combination of cardio and strength training to create a calorie deficit and build muscle, which boosts metabolism.
- **Sample Daily Routine:**
    - Warm-up (5 minutes of light cardio and dynamic stretches).
    - High-Intensity Interval Training (HIIT) Circuit (explained below).
    - 3 sets of this circuit with 1-minute rest periods between sets.
    - Cool-down (5 minutes of light cardio and static stretches).
- **HIIT Circuit:** Perform each exercise for 30 seconds at maximum effort, followed by 15 seconds of rest:
    - Jumping Jacks
    - Mountain Climbers
    - Squat Jumps
    - Burpees (Modification: plank jumps if needed)

Increasing Flexibility:

- **Focus:** Gentle stretches that improve

your range of motion and reduce muscle stiffness.

- **Sample Daily Routine:**
    - 10-15 minute Yoga routine focusing on stretches for major muscle groups (online resources or yoga classes can guide you).
    - Hold each stretch for 20-30 seconds and breathe deeply.
- **Progression:** Gradually increase the hold time for each stretch as your flexibility improves.

Remember:

- These are just sample routines. You can adjust them based on your preferences and fitness level.
- Consult a doctor before starting any new exercise program, especially if you have any health concerns.
- Consistency is key! Aim for at least 30 minutes of moderate-intensity exercise most days of the week.

Chapter 8: Staying Motivated and Tracking Your Progress:

Motivation is the fuel that propels you towards your weight loss goals. This chapter equips you with strategies to stay fired up, track your progress effectively, and use data to stay on track and celebrate your achievements.

Staying Motivated:

Find Your Exercise Tribe: Exercising with a friend or joining a fitness class can boost accountability, make workouts more fun, and provide valuable support.

Reward Yourself: Set healthy rewards for reaching milestones, like a new workout outfit, a massage, or a fun activity.

Set SMART Goals: Specific, Measurable, Achievable, Relevant, and Time-bound goals keep you motivated and focused. Celebrate small victories along the way.

Focus on Progress, Not Perfection: Don't get discouraged by setbacks. Focus on the overall progress you're making and celebrate how far you've come.

Visualize Your Success: Take a moment each day to visualize yourself achieving your goals. This positive reinforcement keeps you motivated.

Tracking Your Progress:

Weight Loss Journals: Maintain a journal to track your weight, measurements, workouts, and how you feel. Seeing your progress written down is a great motivator.

Fitness Trackers: These wearable devices track your steps, calories burned, and activity levels. Use this data to stay accountable and adjust your workouts as needed.

Progress Photos: Take photos of yourself at the beginning of your journey and periodically throughout. Seeing physical changes can be a powerful motivator.

Using Data to Stay on Track:

Monitor Your Weight: Weigh yourself regularly (once a week is sufficient) to monitor trends, but don't become fixated on the number.

Analyze Your Workouts: Track your workout details (exercises, sets, reps, weights) to see your progress and adjust your routine for continued improvement.

Celebrate Non-Scale Victories: Focus on improvements in your energy levels, strength, endurance, and mood, not just the number on the scale.

Make Adjustments: Use the data you collect to adjust your calorie intake or exercise program if needed to stay on track towards your goals.

Staying motivated is a journey, not a destination. There will be ups and downs. Use the strategies in this chapter to keep yourself fired up, track your progress, and celebrate your achievements.

By embracing the data and focusing on positive changes, you'll be well on your way to reaching your weight loss goals and transforming your life through daily exercise.

Part 3

Beyond the Exercises: Maintaining a Healthy Lifestyle

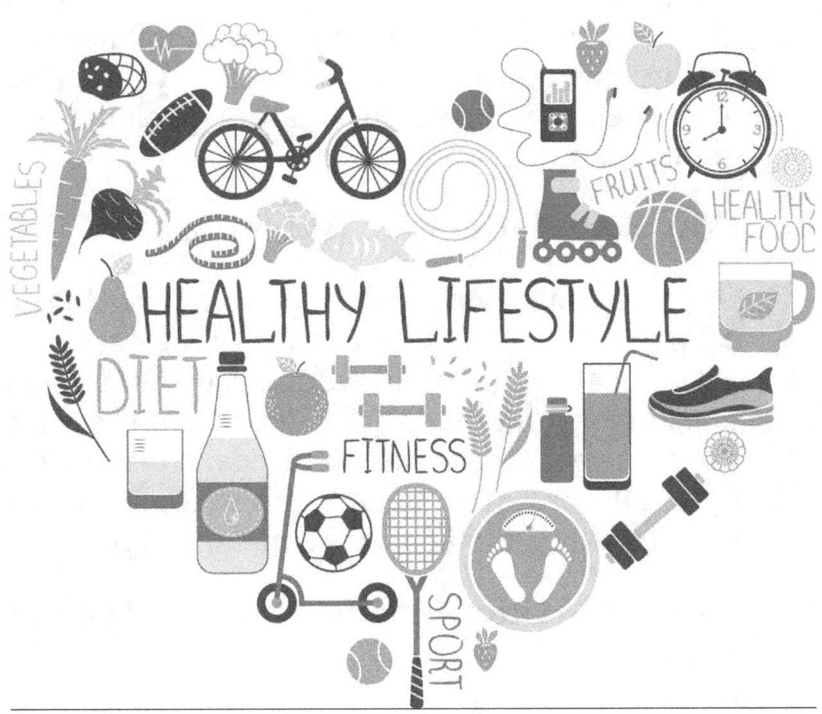

Chapter 9: The Power of Healthy Eating:

Exercise is a crucial pillar for weight loss, but it's not the whole story. To achieve sustainable weight loss and optimal health, you need to combine exercise with a healthy diet. This chapter dives into the importance of healthy eating, introduces basic nutrition principles, and offers resources to create a personalized eating plan.

Why Diet Matters for Weight Loss:

Imagine your body as a car. Exercise burns calories (fuel), but if you keep filling the tank with junk food (inefficient fuel), weight loss will be slow or nonexistent. A healthy diet provides the nutrients your body needs to function optimally, recover from exercise, and build muscle, which further boosts metabolism.

Basic Nutrition Principles for Weight Loss:

- **Portion Control:** Use smaller plates, measuring cups, and mindful eating practices to avoid overeating.

- **Focus on Whole Foods:** Prioritize whole, unprocessed foods like fruits, vegetables, whole grains, lean protein, and healthy fats. These are nutrient-dense and keep you feeling fuller for longer.
- **Limit Processed Foods:** Processed foods are often high in calories, unhealthy fats, sugar, and sodium, offering minimal nutritional value.
- **Stay Hydrated:** Drink plenty of water throughout the day to stay hydrated, support digestion, and curb cravings.

Building a Healthy Eating Plan:

Creating a sustainable eating plan is key. Here are some resources to get you started:

- **Consult a Registered Dietitian:** A registered dietitian can create a personalized plan that considers your preferences, health conditions, and weight loss goals.
- **Online Resources:** Reputable websites and apps offer healthy meal plans and recipes. Choose resources that promote balanced nutrition and avoid fad diets.
- **Books and Magazines:** Numerous books and magazines offer guidance on healthy eating for weight loss. Look for

publications with credible sources and evidence-based information.

Do not forget:

- A healthy diet is not about deprivation. It's about making sustainable choices that nourish your body and fuel your weight loss journey.
- Don't be afraid to experiment and find healthy foods you enjoy. This makes sticking to your eating plan much easier.
- Allow yourself occasional treats in moderation. Rigid restrictions can lead to cravings and binge eating.

Chapter 10: Rest and Recovery:

Your weight loss journey isn't just about burning calories; it's also about giving your body the rest and recovery it needs to thrive. This chapter highlights the importance of rest and recovery for muscle repair, injury prevention, and overall well-being.

Why Rest and Recovery Matter:

- **Muscle Repair:** During exercise, microscopic tears occur in your muscle fibers. Rest allows your body to repair this damage, leading to stronger muscles. Without proper recovery, these tears can worsen, hindering progress and increasing the risk of injuries.
- **Injury Prevention:** Overtraining your body can lead to overuse injuries like muscle strains, tendonitis, and stress fractures. Taking rest days allows your body to rebuild and reduces the risk of such injuries.
- **Improved Performance:** Proper rest and recovery allows your body to replenish energy stores, improve focus,

and enhance your performance during workouts.

Essential Recovery Techniques:

- **Sleep:** Aim for 7-9 hours of quality sleep each night. Sleep is crucial for muscle repair, hormone regulation, and overall physical and mental recovery.
- **Active Recovery:** These low-intensity activities like light cardio, yoga, or stretching promote blood flow, remove waste products, and improve flexibility, aiding in muscle recovery.
- **Stretching:** Regular stretching improves flexibility, reduces muscle soreness, and helps prevent injuries. Stretch both before and after workouts, focusing on major muscle groups.
- **Foam Rolling:** This self-massage technique can help release muscle tension and improve blood flow, promoting recovery.
- **Listen to Your Body:** Pay attention to your body's signals. If you experience excessive fatigue, pain, or decreased motivation, take a rest day or adjust your workout intensity. Pushing yourself through pain can lead to injury and hinder your progress.

Creating a Rest and Recovery Routine:

- **Schedule Rest Days:** Plan rest days into your weekly workout routine. Aim for at least one or two rest days per week, depending on your exercise intensity and experience level.
- **Listen to Your Body:** Don't be afraid to adjust your workout schedule or take an extra rest day if you're feeling overly tired or sore.
- **Prioritize Sleep:** Develop healthy sleep habits like establishing a regular sleep schedule, creating a relaxing bedtime routine, and avoiding screens before bed.
- **Active Recovery Activities:** Incorporate activities like yoga, light walks, or gentle stretching into your rest days to aid recovery.

Remember:

Rest and recovery are not signs of weakness; they are essential components of a successful weight loss and fitness journey. By prioritizing rest, you'll ensure your body has the time and resources it needs to repair, rebuild, and perform at its best, propelling you towards your weight loss goals and a healthier you.

Chapter 11: Building a Healthy Lifestyle:

Congratulations! You've explored the fundamentals of exercise, healthy eating, and rest & recovery. This chapter emphasizes the importance of a holistic approach to weight loss, incorporating strategies beyond diet and exercise that address stress management and building a supportive environment for long-term success.

Why Go Beyond Exercise and Diet?

Weight loss is a multifaceted journey. While exercise and diet are crucial, other factors like stress, sleep, and emotional well-being significantly impact your progress.

- **Stress and Weight Gain:** Chronic stress elevates cortisol levels, a hormone that can promote fat storage, particularly around the belly. Managing stress is essential for regulating your hormones and supporting weight loss efforts.
- **Sleep and Weight Loss:** Poor sleep disrupts hormones that regulate hunger and satiety, leading to increased cravings

and potential overeating. Prioritizing quality sleep is vital for weight management.

- **Emotional Well-being:** Emotional eating can be a coping mechanism for stress or negative emotions. Addressing emotional well-being can help break unhealthy eating patterns and promote sustainable weight loss.

Holistic Strategies for Weight Loss Success:

- **Stress Management Techniques:**
    - **Meditation:** Regular meditation practice reduces stress hormones and promotes relaxation, aiding in weight management.
    - **Deep Breathing Exercises:** Simple deep breathing techniques can calm the nervous system and manage stress in the moment.
    - **Yoga:** Yoga combines physical postures, breathing exercises, and meditation, promoting relaxation and stress reduction.
- **Prioritizing Sleep:** As discussed in Chapter 10, aim for 7-9 hours of quality sleep each night. Develop healthy sleep habits for better sleep hygiene.

- **Building a Positive Support System:** Surround yourself with supportive friends and family who encourage your healthy lifestyle choices. Consider joining a weight loss support group or finding an accountability partner.
- **Mindful Eating:** Practice mindful eating, focusing on the taste, texture, and satiety cues of your food. This promotes controlled portion sizes and helps you avoid mindless overeating.
- **Addressing Emotional Eating:** Identify emotional triggers for unhealthy eating habits. Seek professional help if needed to develop healthier coping mechanisms for stress and negative emotions.

Remember:

A holistic approach to weight loss acknowledges that you are a whole person, not just a body. By addressing all aspects of your well-being, you create a sustainable foundation for weight loss and overall health.

Chapter 12: Conclusion and Looking Forward:

You've come a long way! Take a moment to celebrate your achievements – you've built healthy habits, increased your fitness level, and are well on your way to achieving your weight loss goals. This chapter highlights the importance of lifelong healthy habits, offers tips to prevent weight regain, and inspires you to continue your amazing fitness journey.

Celebrating Your Progress:

- **Acknowledge Your Achievements:** Take time to reflect on how far you've come. Celebrate milestones, big or small, and be proud of your dedication and hard work.
- **Reward Yourself:** Indulge in healthy rewards for reaching goals, like a new workout outfit, a relaxing massage, or a fun activity you enjoy.
- **Focus on How You Feel:** Notice how your exercise routine has positively impacted your energy levels, mood, and overall well-being. Celebrate these non-scale victories.

Embracing Lifelong Healthy Habits:

- **Sustainability is Key:** The goal is to create healthy habits you can maintain for life, not just a quick fix. Focus on making small, sustainable changes you can stick with in the long term.
- **Find Activities You Enjoy:** Exercise shouldn't feel like a chore. Choose activities you genuinely enjoy, making your workouts something you look forward to.
- **Make Healthy Eating a Lifestyle:** Don't restrict yourself excessively. Focus on building a healthy relationship with food, enjoying nutritious meals, and creating a sustainable eating pattern for life.

Preventing Weight Regain:

- **Maintain Your Routine:** Don't abandon your exercise routine and healthy eating habits once you reach your goal weight. Consistency is key to long-term weight management.
- **Adjust as Needed:** Your needs may change over time. Be flexible and adjust your exercise routine and diet to maintain a healthy weight as your life evolves.

- **Listen to Your Body:** Pay attention to your hunger and fullness cues. Don't deprive yourself, but avoid overeating.
- **Seek Support:** Maintain your support system of friends, family, or a weight loss support group for continued motivation and accountability.

The Journey Continues:

This book is just the beginning of your amazing fitness journey. You've equipped yourself with the knowledge and tools to achieve your weight loss goals and live a healthier, happier life. Remember, there will be setbacks along the way.

Don't get discouraged – view them as learning experiences and use them to stay motivated and get back on track. Embrace the journey, celebrate your progress, and continue to inspire yourself and others as you move forward on your path to lifelong health and well-being.

Bonus Chapter : Sample Meal Plans

These are just sample meal plans to give you an idea of how to incorporate healthy eating principles into your daily routine. Remember, portion sizes and specific foods will vary depending on your individual needs and calorie goals. Be sure to consult a doctor or registered dietitian for personalized guidance.

Sample Meal Plan 1 (1500 Calories):

- **Breakfast (400 calories):**
    - Greek yogurt with berries and a sprinkle of granola
- **Lunch (500 calories):**
    - Grilled chicken breast salad with mixed greens, vegetables, and a light vinaigrette dressing
    - Whole-wheat bread or brown rice
- **Snack (200 calories):**
    - Apple slices with almond butter
- **Dinner (400 calories):**
    - Salmon with roasted vegetables and quinoa

Sample Meal Plan 2 (1800 Calories):

- **Breakfast (450 calories):**
  - Whole-wheat oatmeal with nuts and seeds
- **Lunch (550 calories):**
  - Lentil soup with a whole-wheat roll
  - Side salad with a light vinaigrette dressing
- **Snack (200 calories):**
  - Cottage cheese with chopped vegetables
- **Dinner (600 calories):**
  - Turkey stir-fry with brown rice and vegetables

Sample Meal Plan 3 (2000 Calories):

- **Breakfast (500 calories):**
  - Scrambled eggs with whole-wheat toast and avocado
- **Lunch (600 calories):**
  - Tuna salad sandwich on whole-wheat bread with a side salad
  - Light yogurt with fruit
- **Snack (200 calories):**

- o Handful of mixed nuts and dried fruit
- **Dinner (700 calories):**
  - o Chicken breast with roasted sweet potato and broccoli

Tips:

- Aim for at least 3 meals and 2-3 snacks per day to keep your metabolism fueled and prevent overeating.
- Include plenty of fruits, vegetables, and whole grains in your diet for essential vitamins, minerals, and fiber.
- Choose lean protein sources like chicken, fish, beans, or lentils to feel satisfied and support muscle building.
- Limit unhealthy fats, processed foods, sugary drinks, and added sugars.
- Drink plenty of water throughout the day to stay hydrated.

These are just samples. There are endless possibilities for creating healthy and delicious meals that fit your preferences and calorie goals. Be creative, explore new recipes, and find what works best for you on your weight loss journey!